To my husband, thank you for believing in me.

To my friends and family, thank you for supporting me.

To our future child, you are already so loved.

Everyone is unique;

families are too.

How your family is made

may not be up to you.

Some families have one parent;

some families have two.

Some families have one mommy or daddy

that equally love you.

Just like families,

the path to making one will be your own.

Know that there is no right or wrong way,

and know that you're not alone.

First there was me,

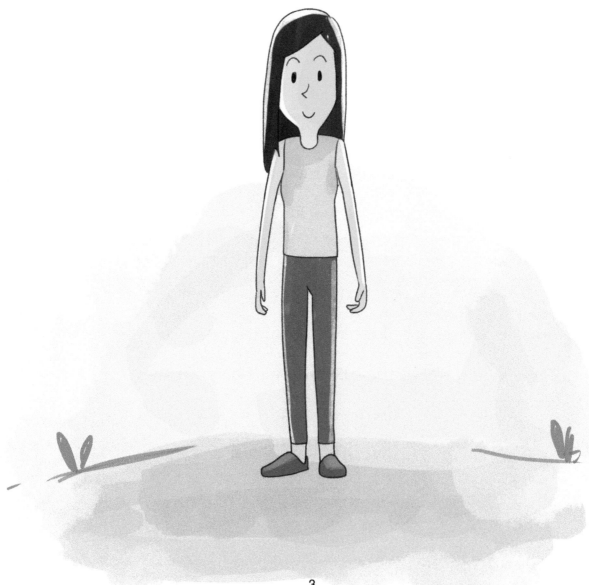

then we.

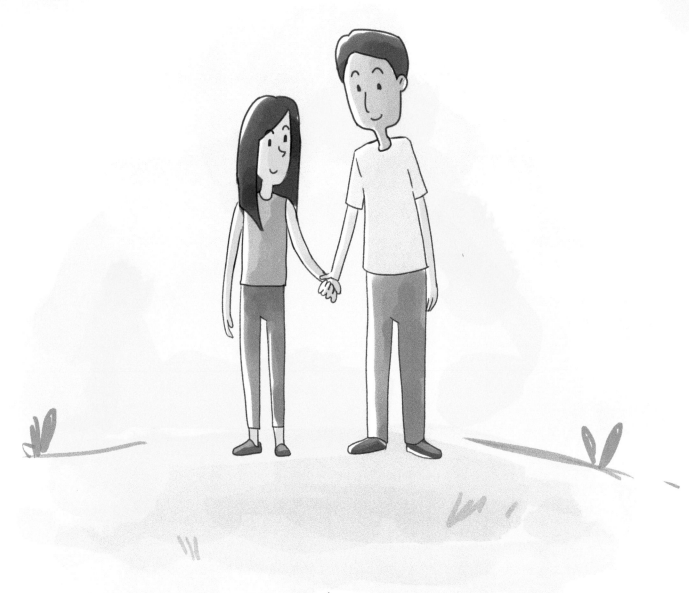

We were two,

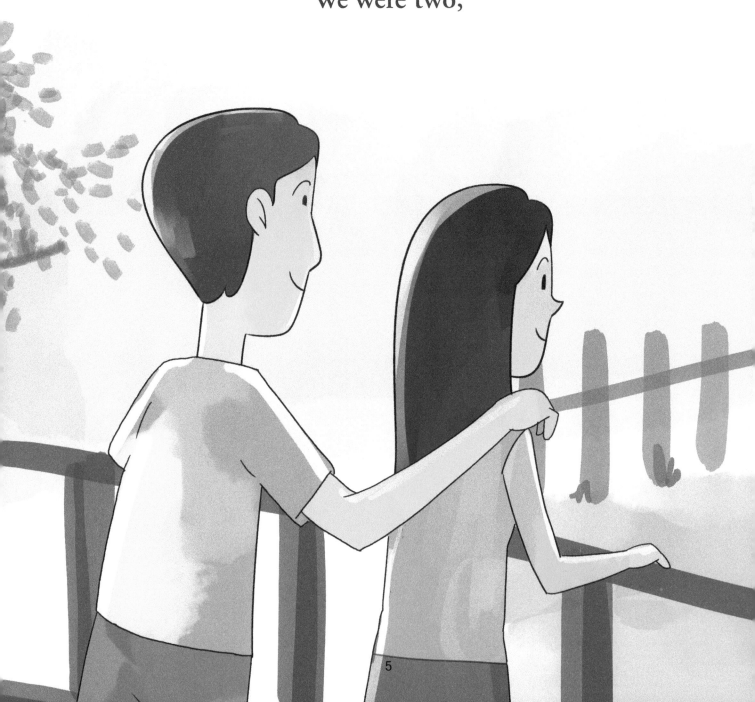

then we were four.

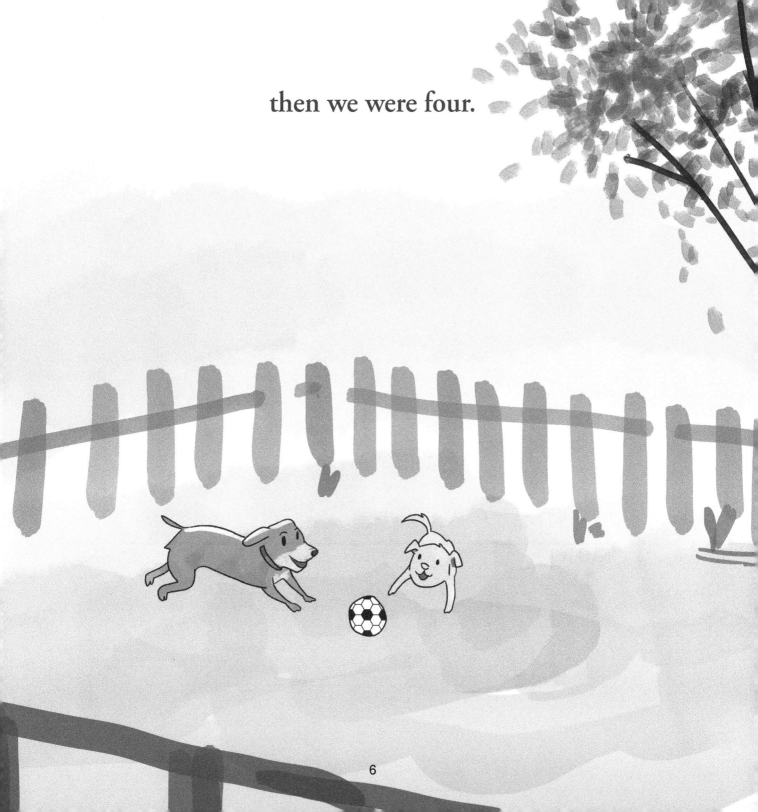

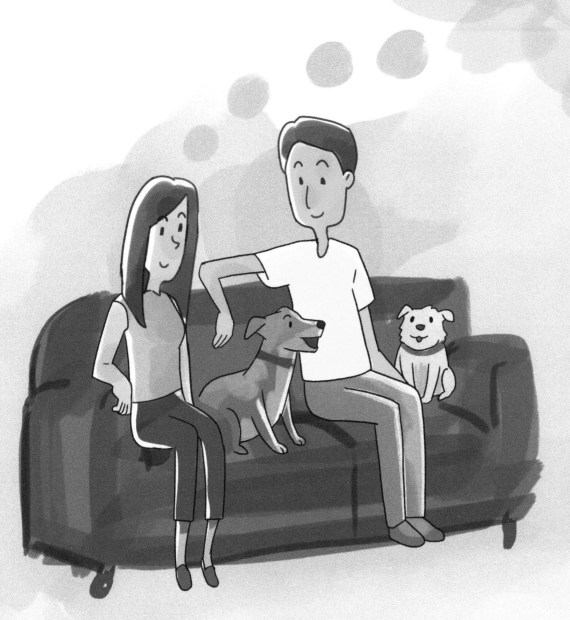

We had so much love in our house,

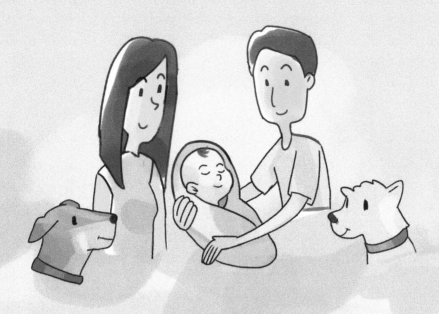

but we wanted more.

We knew a little baby was just what we needed,

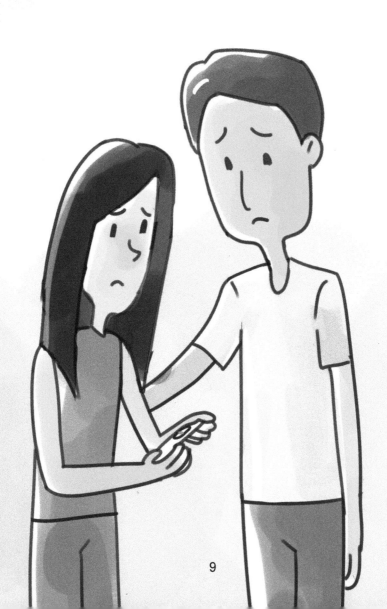

but we weren't expecting the journey that proceeded.

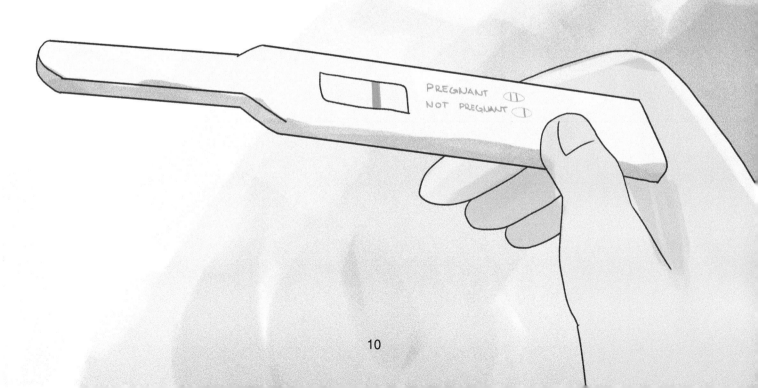

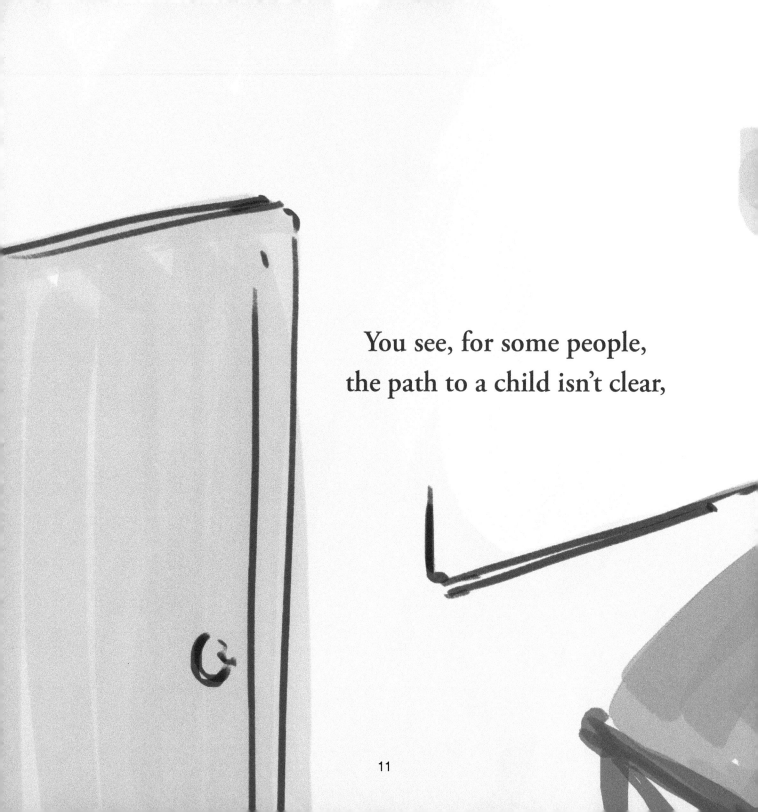

You see, for some people,
the path to a child isn't clear,

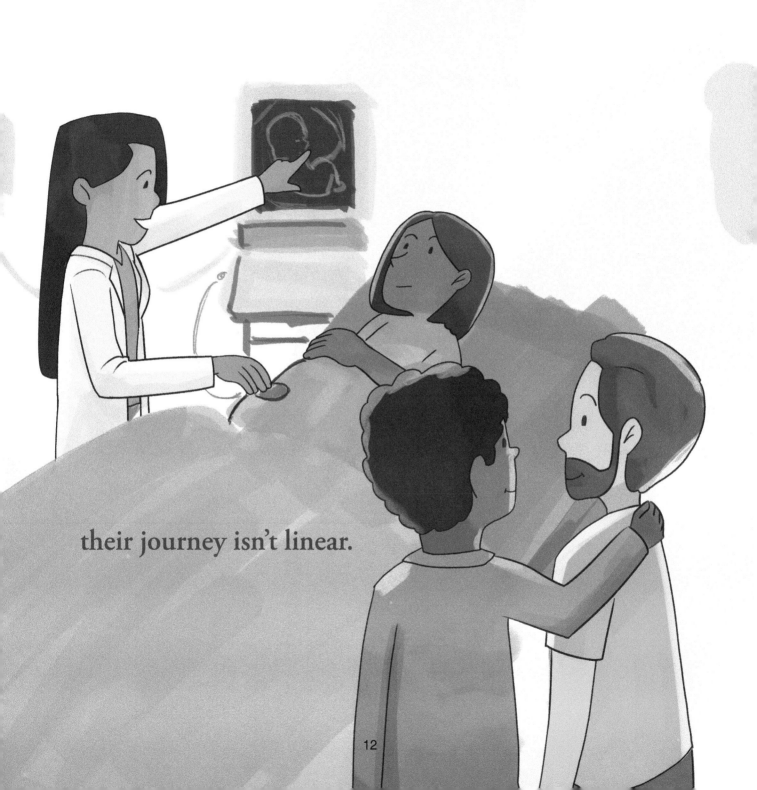

their journey isn't linear.

The process is intimidating,

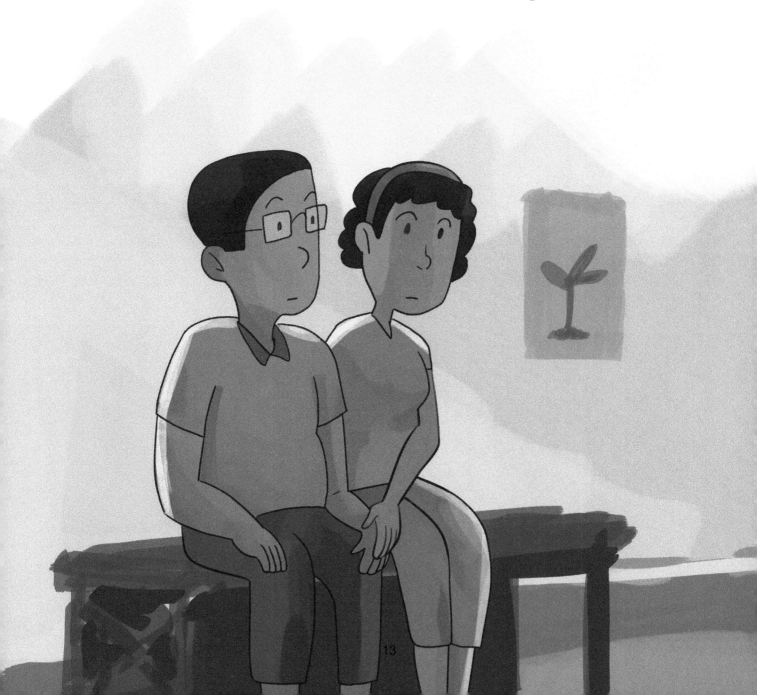

13

and sometimes isolating.

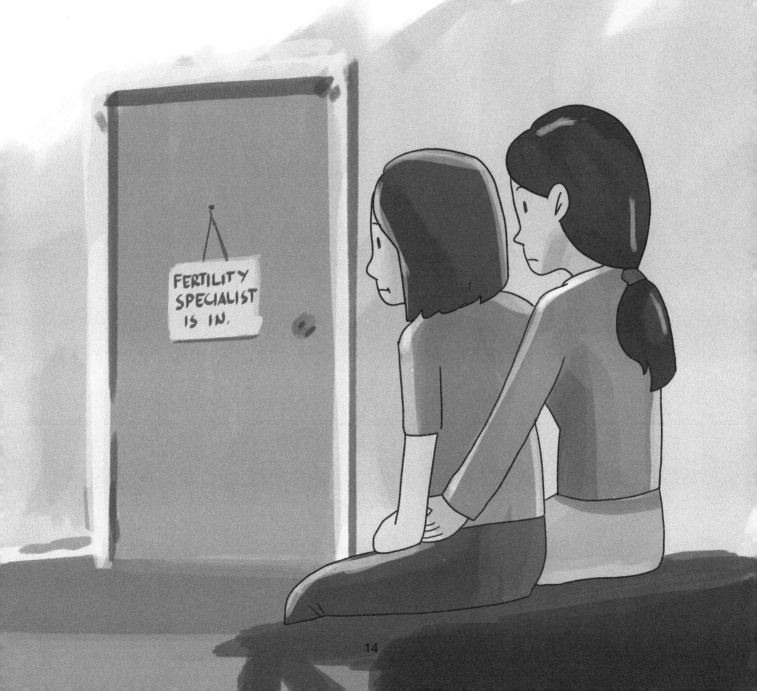

And through this there is no guarantee,

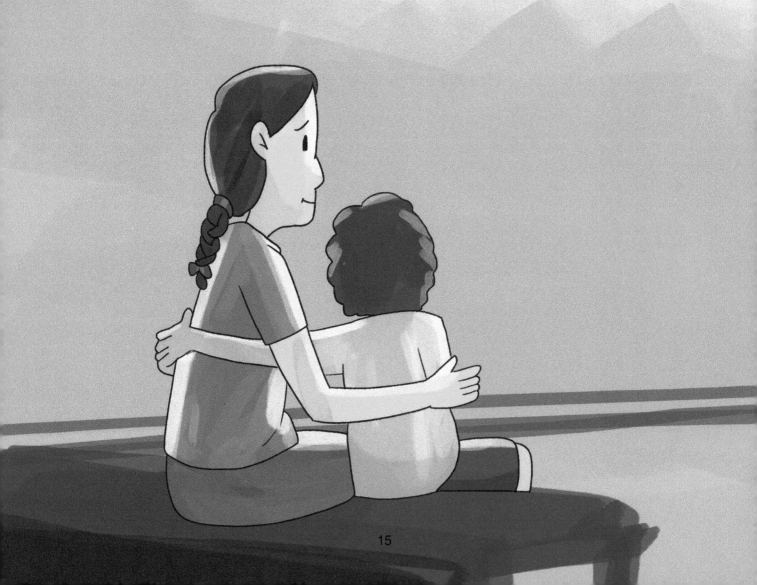

of what the final results will be.

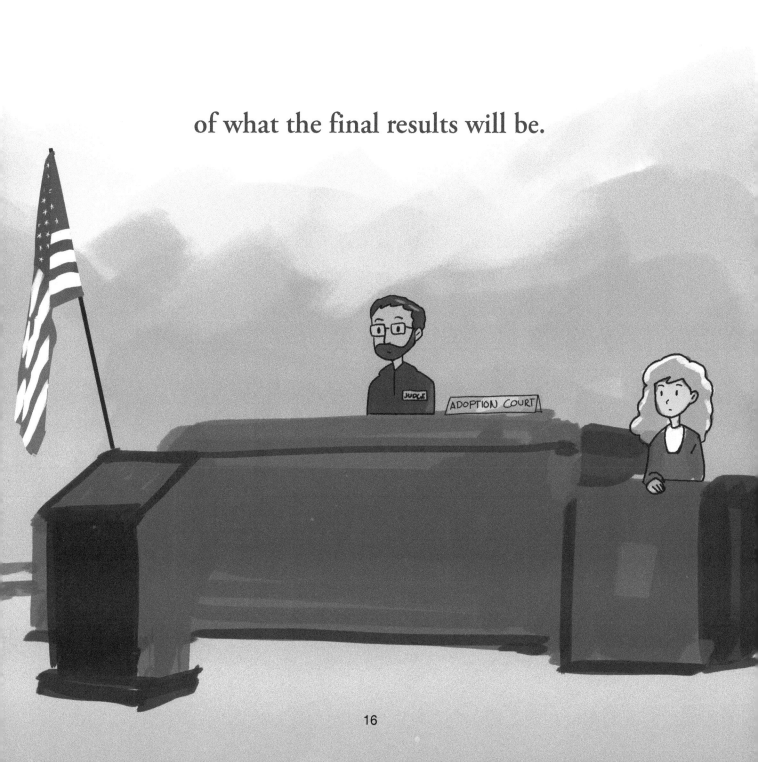

We would go to the ends of the earth for you,

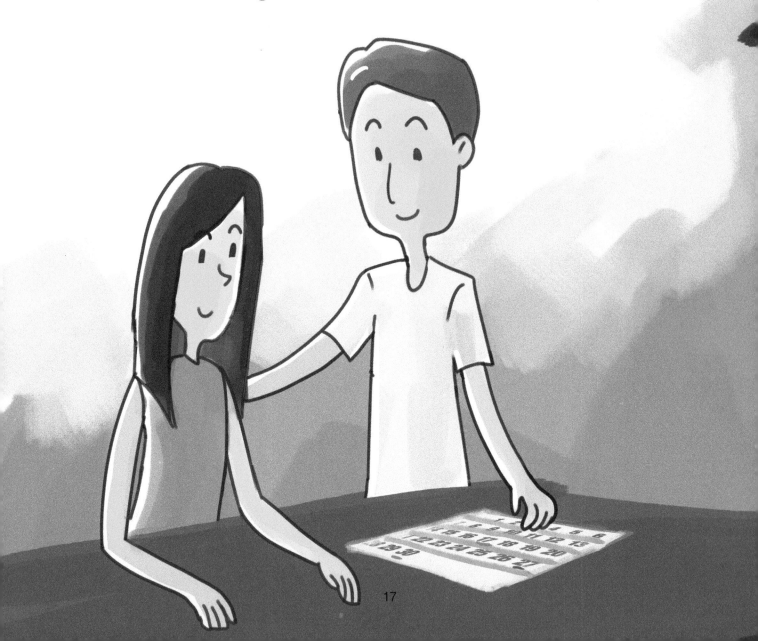

17

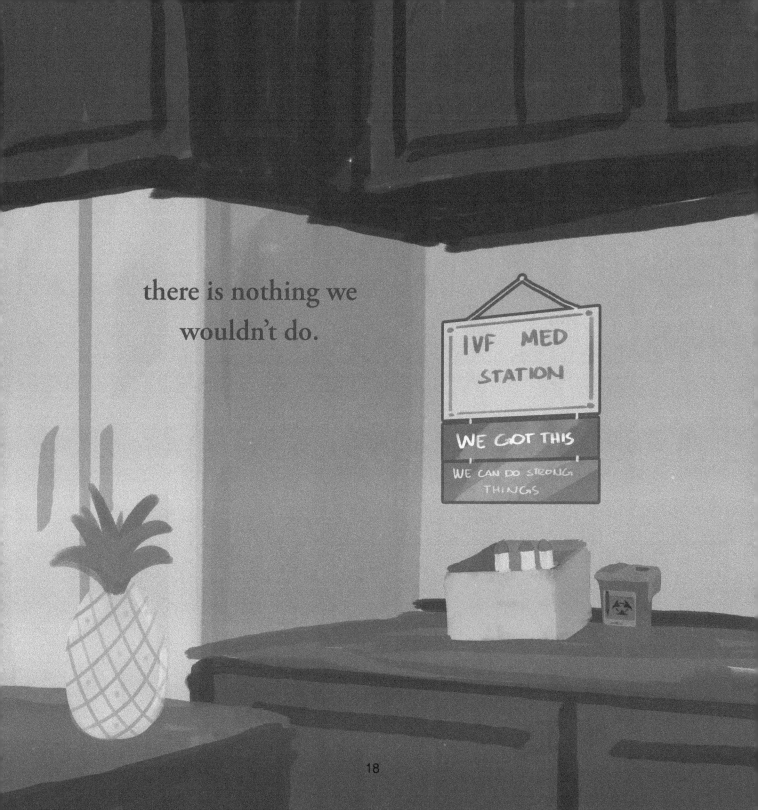

there is nothing we
wouldn't do.

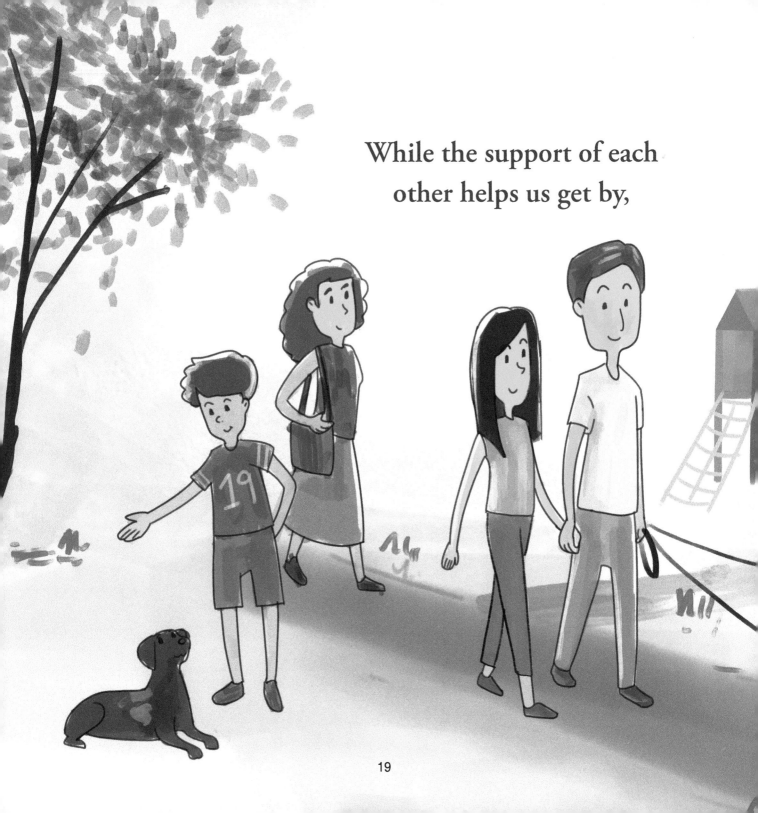

While the support of each
other helps us get by,

we also stay hopeful and keep
our heads held high.

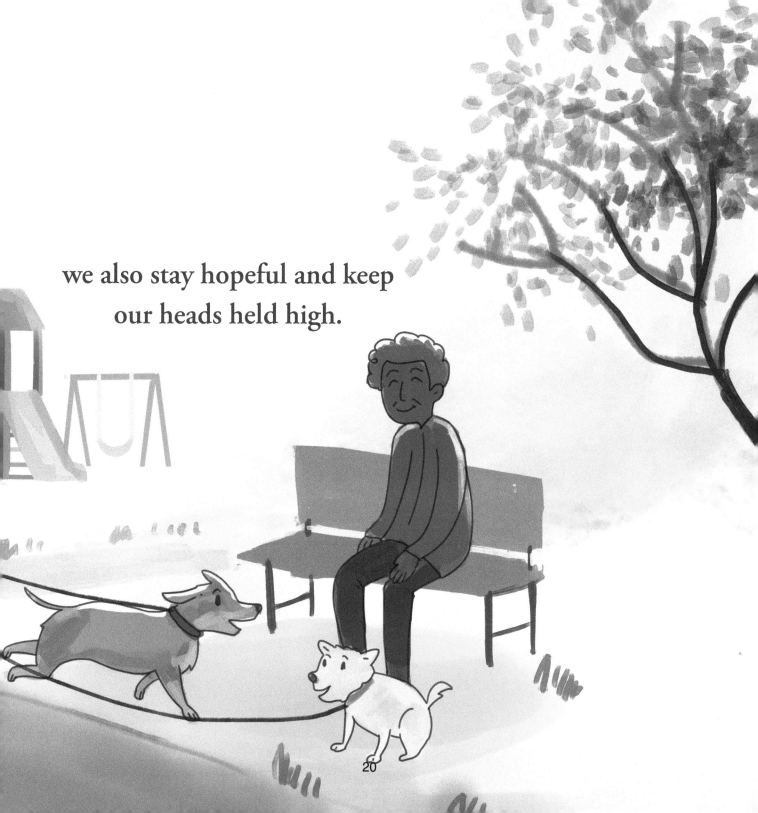

Because our dreams of you are so bright,

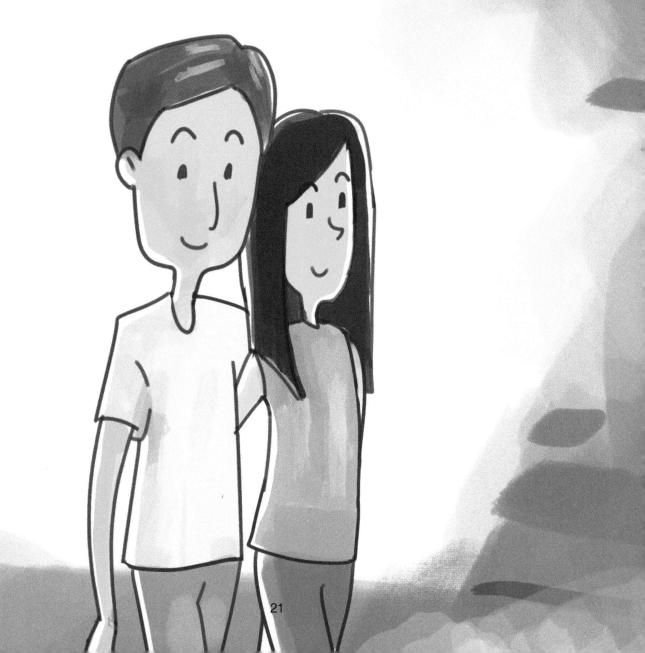

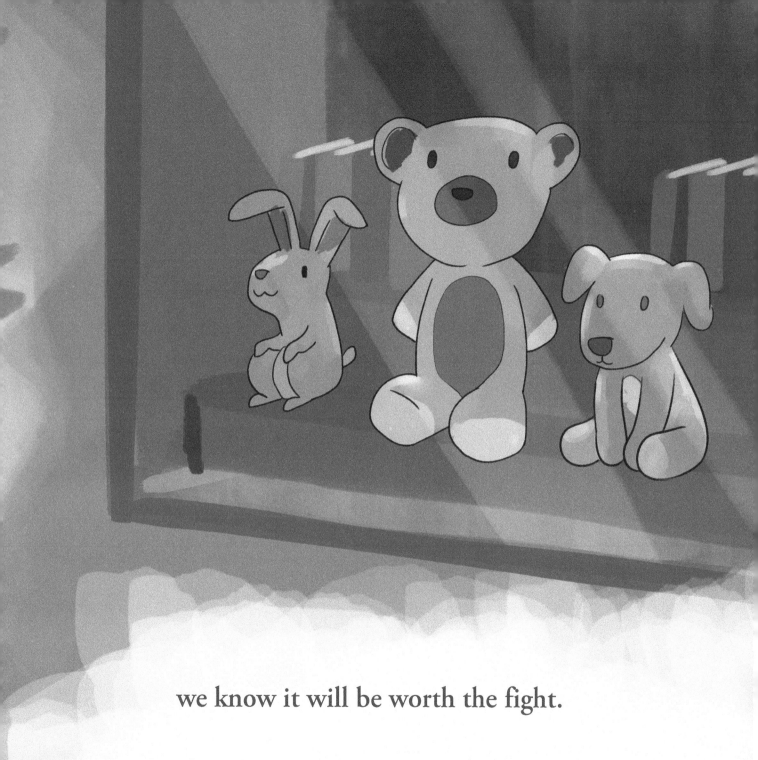

we know it will be worth the fight.

Remember every family starts in its own way,

so love yours to the fullest each and every day.

# About the Author

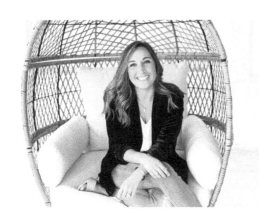

Jaimie Selwa lives with her husband and their two rescued pups in Ohio. She's an active advocate for animal-rescue organizations and a volunteer for local nonprofits.

While helping those organizations find their voice, she found her own in her infertility journey. She and her husband never thought they'd be diagnosed with infertility when they were trying to expand their family. But when life gave her lemons, she decided to make lemonade. She is making it her mission to educate and bring awareness to the many ways you can make a family.

For an honest and humorous look into the life of infertility, follow Jaimie on Instagram at @InfertileChronicles.

CPSIA information can be obtained
at www.ICGtesting.com
Printed in the USA
LVHW071513300721
694156LV00022B/1557

9 781649 524690